Essential Oils for Beginners

A Step-by-Step Guide for Beginners with 25 Recipes

Disclaimer and Terms of Use:

Effort has been made to ensure that the information in this book is accurate and complete, however, the author and the publisher do not warrant the accuracy of the information, text and graphics contained within the book due to the rapidly changing nature of science, research, known and unknown facts and internet. The Author and the publisher do not hold any responsibility for errors, omissions or contrary interpretation of the subject matter herein. This book is presented solely for motivational and informational purposes only.

Table of Contents

Introduction

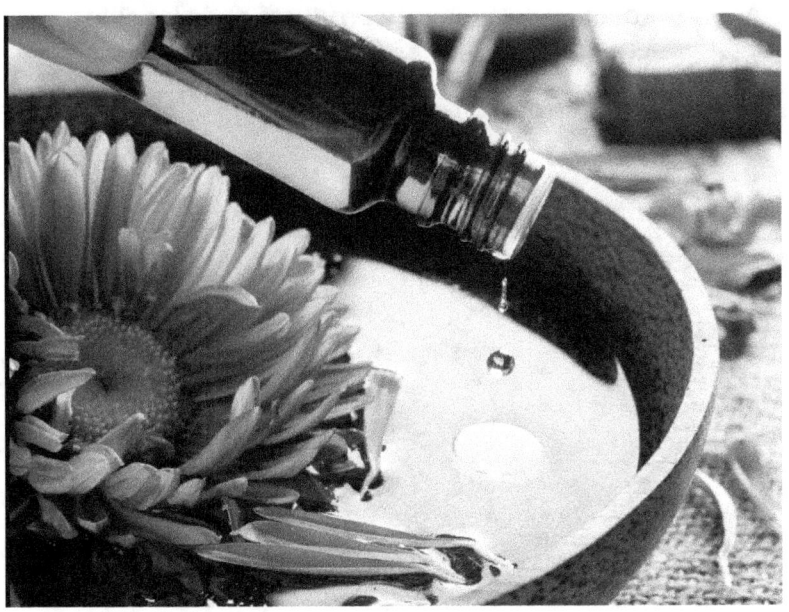

Essential oils are nature's gift to man. They contain the "essence" of the plants from which they are derived, as well as the majority of the beneficial properties contained within the plants. Essential oils have been used for centuries in natural remedies and alternative medicine to treat diseases and various health conditions. In addition to being used for herbal remedies, essential oils can also be used in all-natural beauty products and cleaning supplies.

If you have ever wondered about the benefits of essential oils, this book is the perfect place to begin. In this book you will find a collection of twenty-five essential oil recipes for everything from herbal teas and natural remedies to all-natural beauty products and cleaning supplies. If you are ready to experience the benefits of essential oils for yourself, pick a recipe and get started!

Essential Oils Recipes

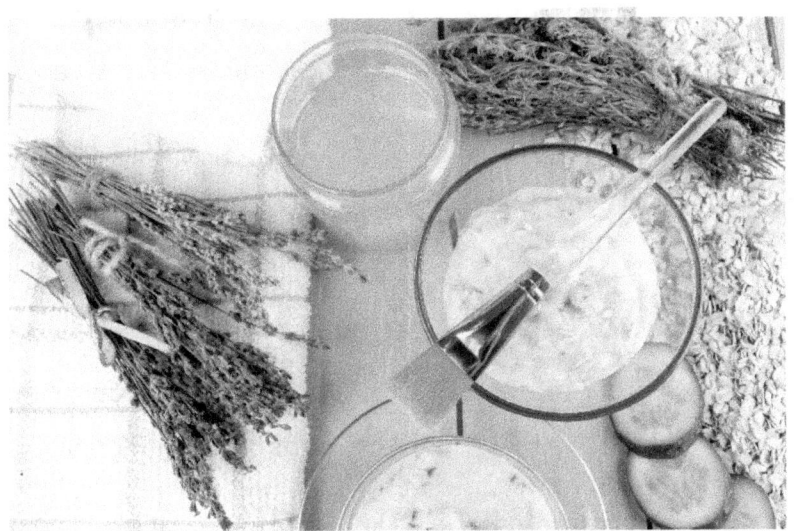

Recipes Included in this Book:

Relaxing Lavender Bath Salts

Lovely Lavender Shampoo

Rosemary Peppermint Shampoo

Perky Peppermint Lip Balm

Whipped Peppermint Body Butter

Stress-Relieving Sugar Scrub

Spiced Maple Lip Balm

Decongestant Chest Rub

Detoxifying Citrus Bath Salts

Warming Cinnamon Lotion Bars

Lemon Lavender Salve

Calming Chamomile
Room Spray

Soothing Eucalyptus
Inhalation

Cold-Stopping Essential
Oil Tea

Cramp-Relieving Clary
Sage Compress

Cheery Grapefruit Air
Freshener

Sinus-Clearing Tea Tree
Inhalation

Migraine Mending
Rosemary Compress

Antiseptic Surface Spray

All-Natural Lemon
Furniture Polish

Lavender Citrus Linen
Spray

Citrus-Scented Carpet
Deodorizer

Garbage Disposal
Cleaning Cubes

Lavender Tea Tree
Laundry Soap

Antiseptic Floor Cleaner

Relaxing Lavender Bath Salts

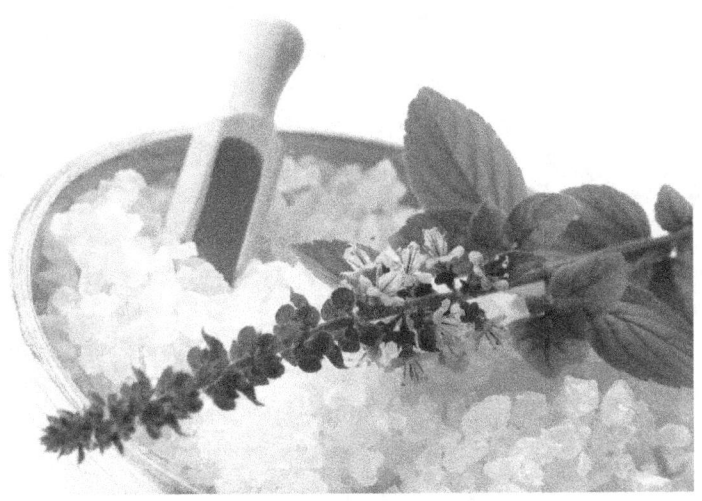

Ingredients:

- 2 cups coarse sea salts
- 1 tablespoon jojoba oil
- 15 drops lavender essential oil
- 10 drops geranium essential oil

Instructions:

1. Place the salt in a medium-sized bowl.
2. Add the jojoba oil and the essential oils then stir well to combine.
3. Store the salts in a glass jar or airtight container.
4. Add ¼ to ½ cup of the salts to running bath water then stir gently by hand.
5. Soak in the bath for at least 30 minutes then towel dry.

Rosemary Peppermint Shampoo

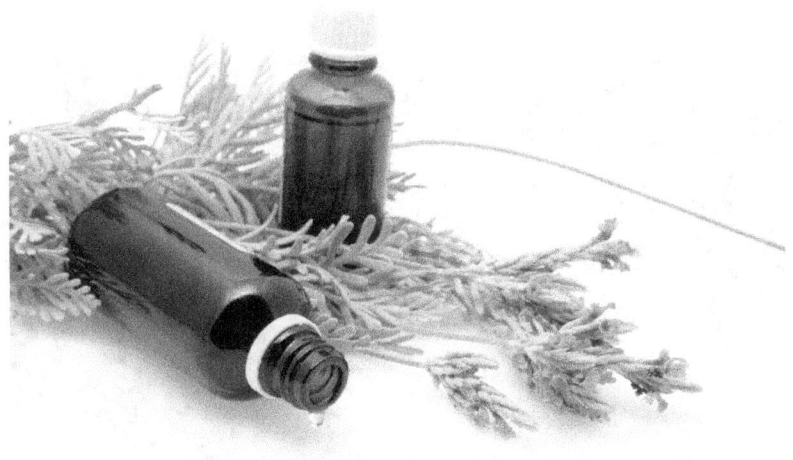

Ingredients:

- ½ cup liquid castile soap, unscented
- 15 drops rosemary essential oil
- 4 drops peppermint essential oil
- ½ cup filtered water

Instructions:

1. Pour the soap into an empty plastic shampoo bottle.
2. Add the essential oils and swirl gently to combine.
3. Pour in the filtered water and shake the bottle gently to combine.
4. Add a small amount of shampoo to damp hair and work into a lather.
5. Rinse your hair completely then towel dry and style as usual.

Whipped Peppermint Body Butter

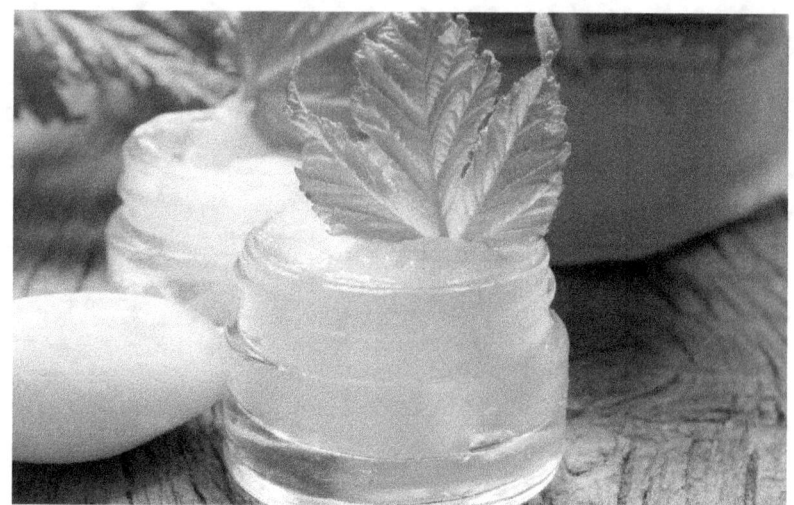

Ingredients:

- ½ cup shea butter
- ½ cup cocoa butter
- ½ cup organic coconut oil
- ½ cup sweet almond oil
- 20 drops peppermint essential oil

Instructions:

1. Combine the shea butter, cocoa butter and coconut oil in a double boiler.
2. Heat until the ingredients are melted then stir smooth.
3. Remove from heat and whisk in the almond oil and essential oils.

4. Pour the mixture into a bowl then chill for 1 hour until it starts to solidify.
5. Beat the mixture with a hand mixer on high speed until fluffy – about 8 to 10 minutes.
6. Place the bowl back in the fridge for 10 minutes then store in a glass jar.

Spiced Maple Lip Balm

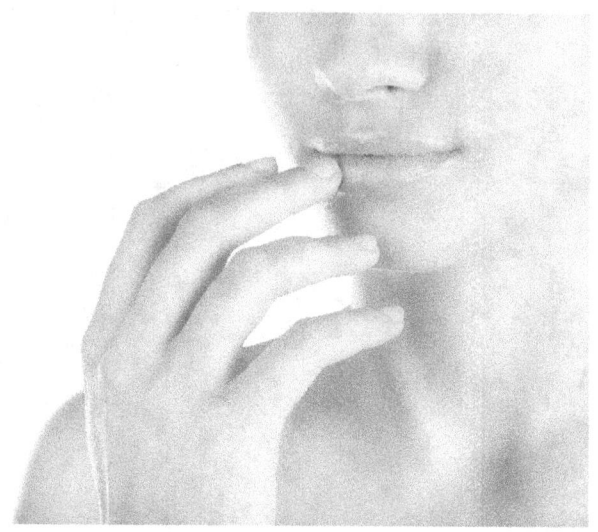

Ingredients:

- 12 empty plastic lip balm tubes
- 2 tablespoons organic coconut oil
- 2 tablespoons beeswax granules
- 1 tablespoon cocoa butter
- ½ teaspoon pure maple syrup
- 3 teaspoons jojoba oil
- 10 drops cinnamon essential oil
- 2 drops clove essential oil
- 2 drops ginger essential oil

Instructions:

1. Combine the coconut oil, beeswax, cocoa butter, and honey in a double boiler.
2. Heat the mixture until melted then remove from heat.

3. Stir in the jojoba oil and essential oils until well combined.
4. Pour the mixture into the lip balm tubes and set them upright.
5. Allow the lip balm to set then put the caps on the tubes and use the balm as needed.

Detoxifying Citrus Bath Salts

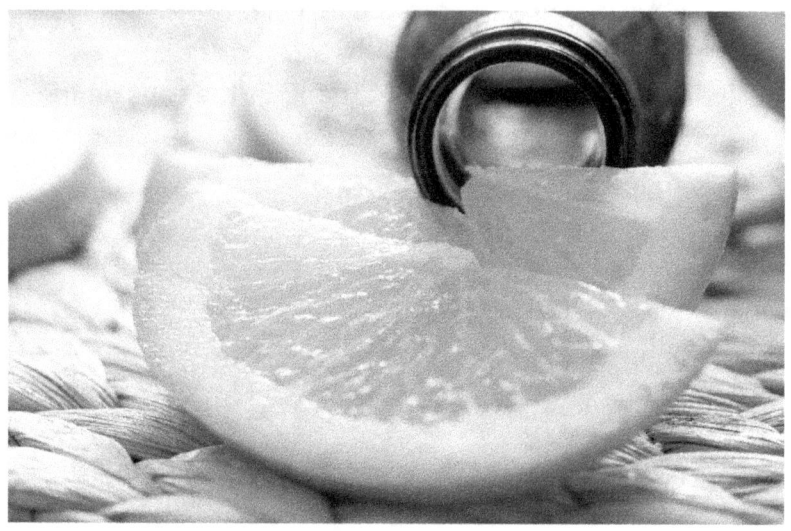

Ingredients:

- 2 cups coarse sea salts
- 1 tablespoon jojoba oil
- 15 drops bergamot essential oil
- 10 drops lemon essential oil
- 5 drops grapefruit essential oil

Instructions:

1. Place the salt in a medium-sized bowl.
2. Add the jojoba oil and the essential oils then stir well to combine.
3. Store the salts in a glass jar or airtight container.
4. Add ¼ to ½ cup of the salts to running bath water then stir gently by hand.
5. Soak in the bath for at least 30 minutes then towel dry.

Lovely Lavender Shampoo

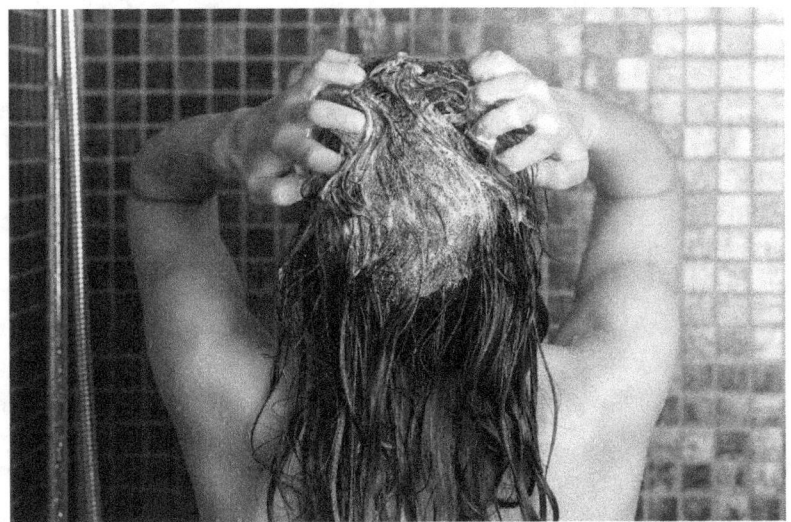

Ingredients:

- ½ cup liquid castile soap, unscented
- 15 drops lavender essential oil
- 4 drops rose essential oil
- ½ cup filtered water

Instructions:

1. Pour the soap into an empty plastic shampoo bottle.
2. Add the essential oils and swirl gently to combine.
3. Pour in the filtered water and shake the bottle gently to combine.
4. Add a small amount of shampoo to damp hair and work into a lather.
5. Rinse your hair completely then towel dry and style as usual.

Perky Peppermint Lip Balm

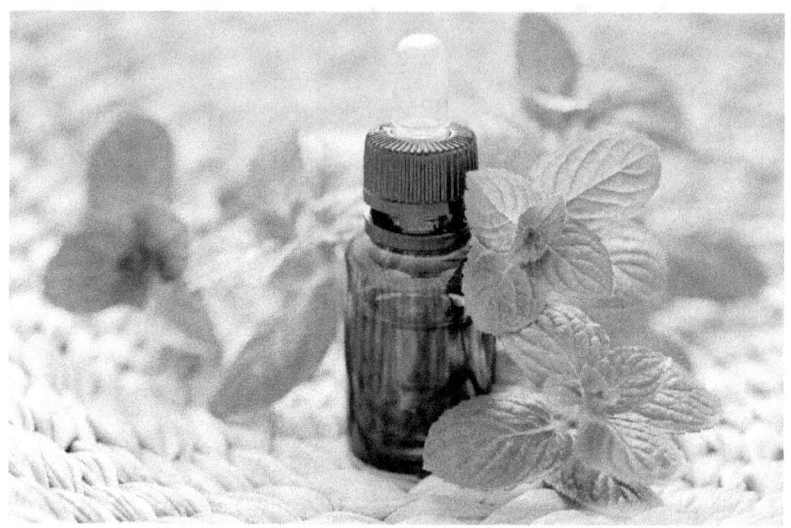

Ingredients:

- 12 empty plastic lip balm tubes
- 2 tablespoons organic coconut oil
- 2 tablespoons beeswax granules
- 1 tablespoon cocoa butter
- ½ teaspoon raw honey
- 3 teaspoons jojoba oil
- 15 drops peppermint essential oil

Instructions:

1. Combine the coconut oil, beeswax, cocoa butter, and honey in a double boiler.
2. Heat the mixture until melted then remove from heat.
3. Stir in the jojoba oil and essential oils until well combined.

4. Pour the mixture into the lip balm tubes and set them upright.
5. Allow the lip balm to set then put the caps on the tubes and use the balm as needed.

Stress-Relieving Sugar Scrub

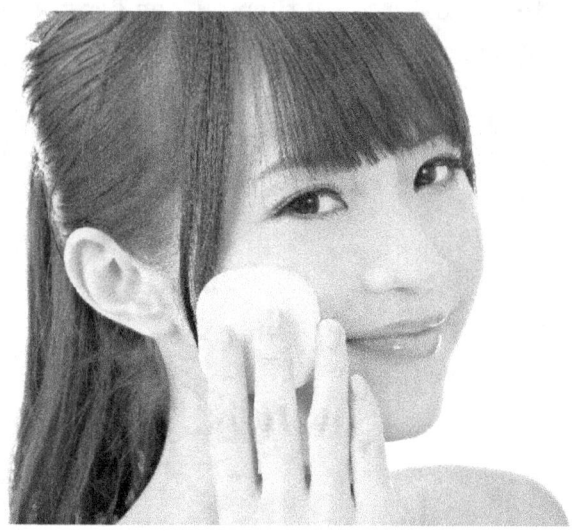

Ingredients:

- 1 cup organic cane sugar
- ¼ cup extra-virgin olive oil
- 2 tablespoons raw honey
- 20 drops lavender essential oil
- 10 drops geranium essential oil
- 10 drops ylang-ylang essential oil

Instructions:

1. Combine the sugar, olive oil and honey in a glass jar.
2. Stir in the essential oils until well combined.
3. Apply a small amount of the scrub to dampened skin.
4. Rub the scrub into your skin to exfoliate and to relieve stress.

Decongestant Chest Rub

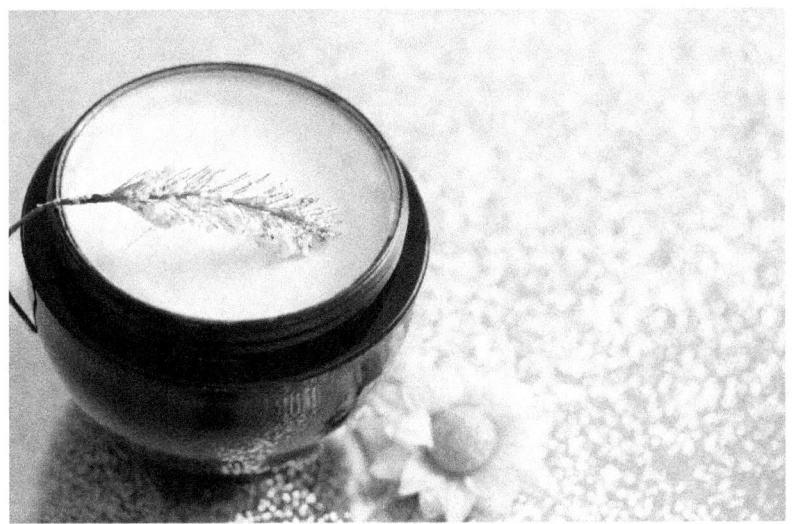

Ingredients:

- ¼ cup organic coconut oil
- 1 ½ tablespoons beeswax granules
- 1 ½ tablespoons jojoba oil
- ½ teaspoon eucalyptus essential oil
- ½ teaspoon lavender essential oil

Instructions:

1. Combine the coconut oil and beeswax in a double boiler until melted.
2. Remove from heat and cool to room temperature.
3. Combine the jojoba oil and essential oils in a small glass jar.
4. Pour in the oil and wax mixture then stir well.
5. Place the jar in the refrigerator until the mixture solidifies.

6. Rub a small amount of the mixture into the skin on your chest to relieve congestion.

Warming Cinnamon Lotion Bars

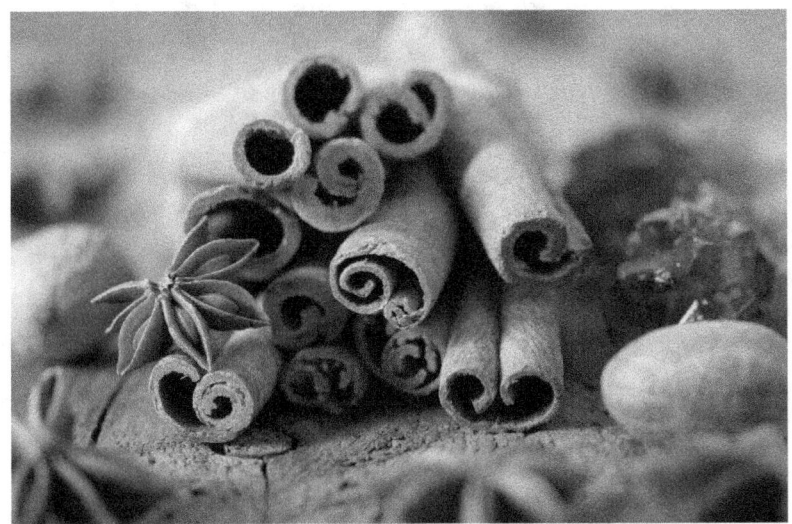

Ingredients:

- ½ cup organic coconut oil
- ½ cup shea butter
- ½ cup beeswax granules
- 20 drops cinnamon essential oil
- 10 drops clove essential oil

Instructions:

1. Combine the coconut oil, shea butter and beeswax in a double boiler.
2. Stir the mixture until melted then stir smooth.
3. Remove from heat and stir in the cinnamon and clove essential oils.
4. Grease a miniature cupcake tin with extra coconut oil.

5. Pour the melted lotion mixture into the tin, filling the cups almost completely.
6. Let the molds set at room temperature until the lotion bars are hardened.
7. To use, rub the lotion bar between your hands to warm it and rub the lotion in.

Lemon Lavender Salve

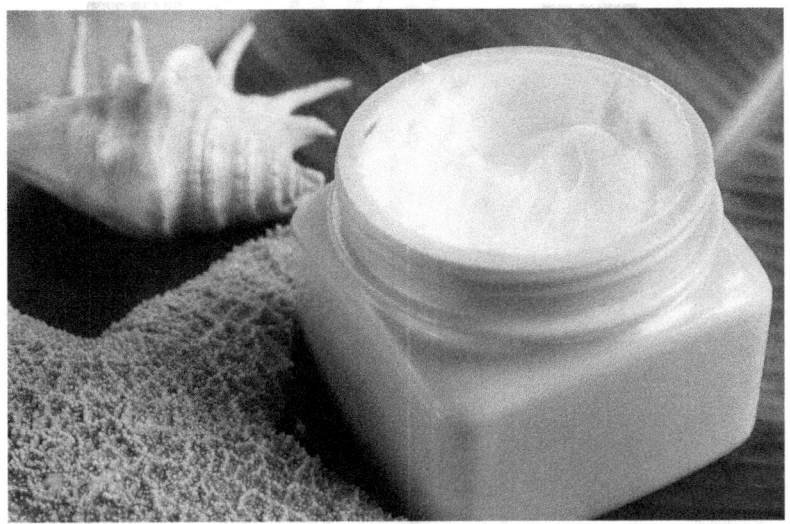

Ingredients:

- 2 tablespoons coconut oil
- 6 drops lemon essential oil
- 6 drops lavender essential oil
- 4 drops tea tree essential oil

Instructions:

1. Place the coconut oil in a small bowl and warm it in the microwave until melted.
2. Add the essential oils and stir until well combined.
3. Pour the mixture into a small glass or metal lotion container.
4. Allow the mixture to sit at room temperature until solidified.
5. Apply the salve directly to your skin as needed to soothe and moisturize.

Calming Chamomile Room Spray

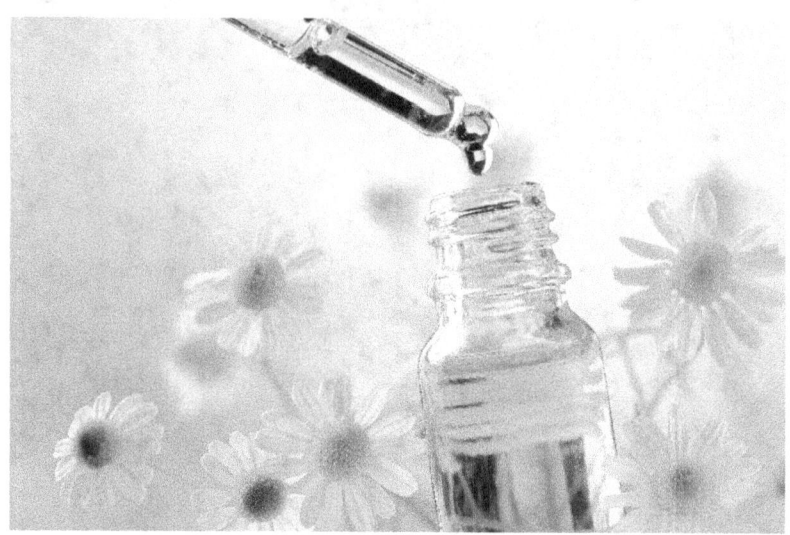

Ingredients:

- Empty 16-ounce plastic spray bottle
- 2 cups filtered water
- 10 drops chamomile essential oil

Instructions:

1. Pour the water into the plastic bottle.
2. Add the chamomile essential oil and shake gently to combine.
3. Spritz the liquid into the air to create a calm and relaxing atmosphere.

Soothing Eucalyptus Inhalation

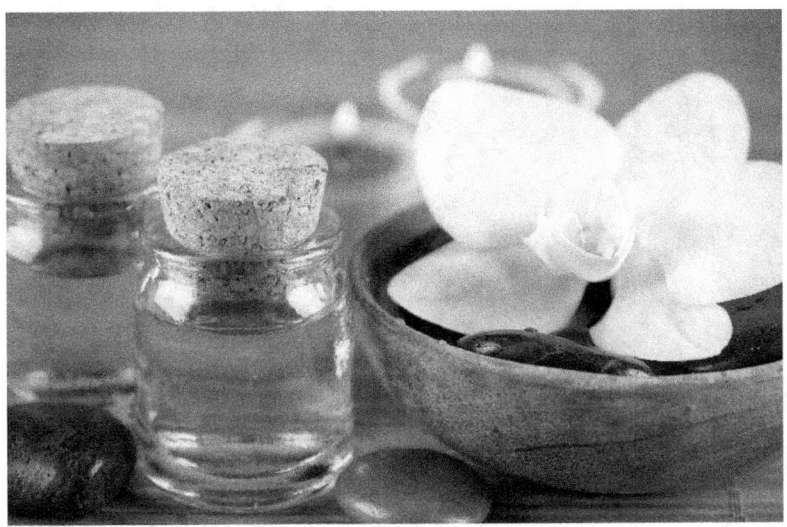

Ingredients:

- Boiling water
- 5 drops eucalyptus essential oil

Instructions:

1. Fill a large bowl with boiling water and place it on a table.
2. Add the eucalyptus oil to the water and stir gently to combine.
3. Sit at the table and lean over the bowl.
4. Cover your head and shoulders with a towel or blanket.
5. Slowly and deeply inhale the steam to relieve symptoms of cold and respiratory illness.

Cold-Stopping Essential Oil Tea

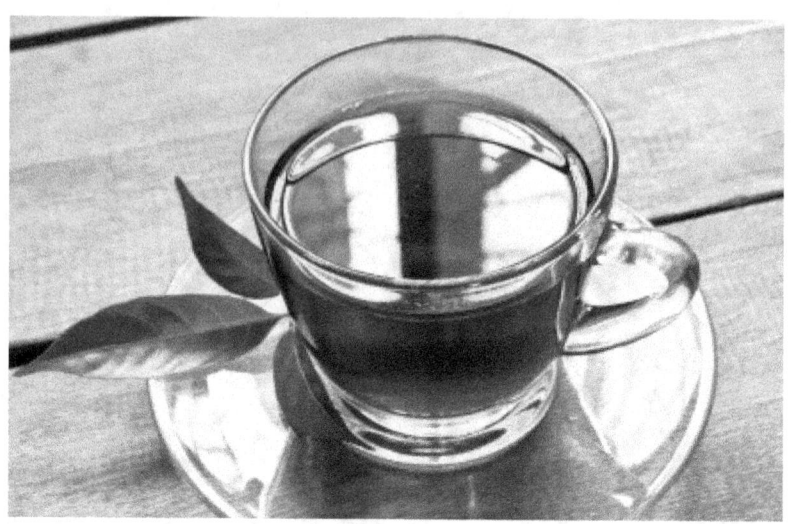

Ingredients:

- 1 teaspoon raw honey
- 2 drops lemon essential oil
- 1 drop thieves essential oil

Instructions:

1. Combine the honey and essentials in a mug.
2. Stir well then pour in the boiling water.
3. Let the tea steep for a minute or two and stir well.
4. Sip the tea slowly to relieve sore throat and cough.

Cramp-Relieving Clary Sage Compress

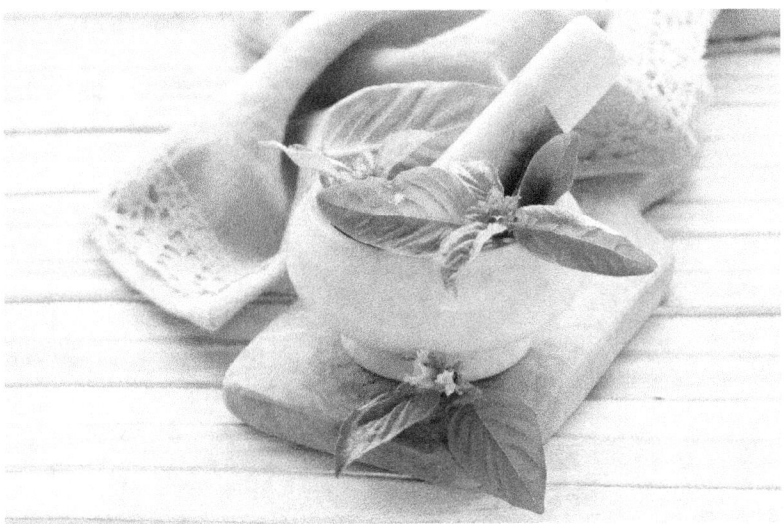

Ingredients:

- Very hot water, as needed
- 5 drops clary sage essential oil
- Clean cotton cloth

Instructions:

1. Fill a medium bowl with very hot water.
2. Add the clary sage essential oils and stir gently.
3. Dip a folded cotton cloth into the hot water and wring out the excess.
4. Place the compress over your abdomen.
5. Let the compress set until it cools to body temperature.

6. Repeat the process three to five times or until your cramps subside.

Cheery Grapefruit Air Freshener

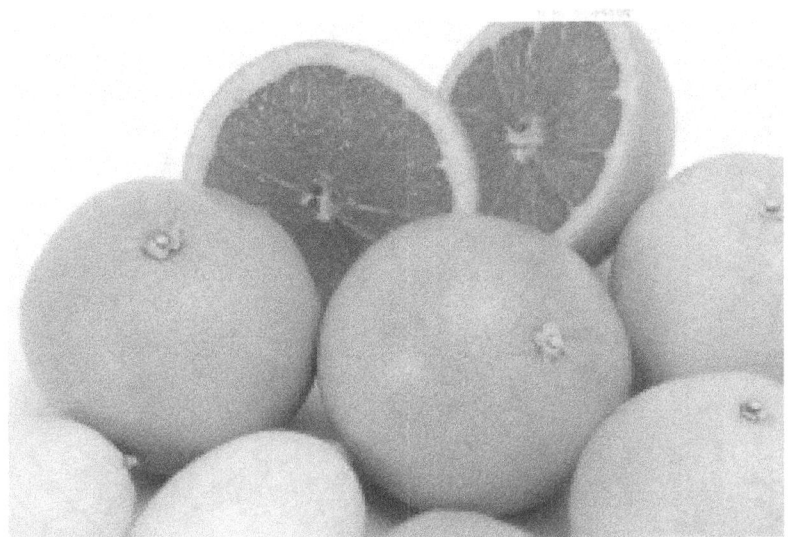

Ingredients:

- Empty 16-ounce plastic spray bottle
- 2 cups filtered water
- 10 drops grapefruit essential oil

Instructions:

1. Pour the water into the plastic bottle.
2. Add the chamomile essential oil and shake gently to combine.
3. Spritz the liquid into the air to create an uplifting and cheerful atmosphere.

Sinus-Clearing Tea Tree Inhalation

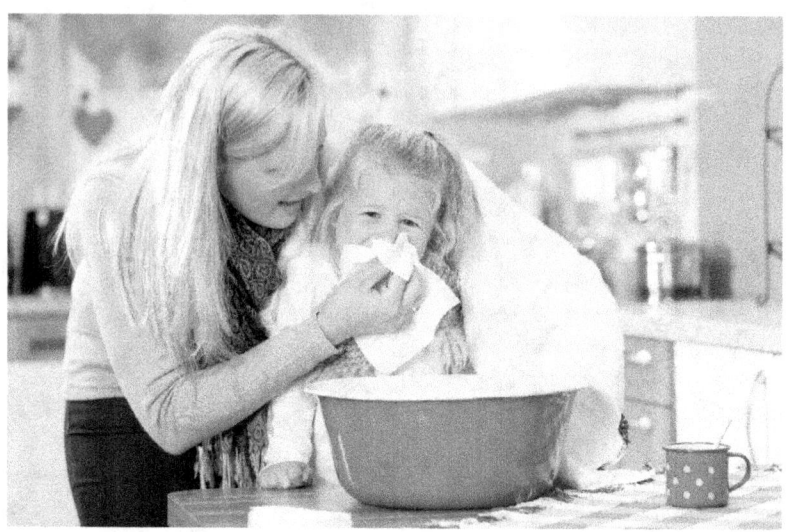

Ingredients:

- Boiling water
- 5 drops tea tree essential oil

Instructions:

1. Fill a large bowl with boiling water and place it on a table.
2. Add the tea tree oil to the water and stir gently to combine.
3. Sit at the table and lean over the bowl.
4. Cover your head and shoulders with a towel or blanket.
5. Slowly and deeply inhale the steam to clear your sinuses.

Migraine Mending Rosemary Compress

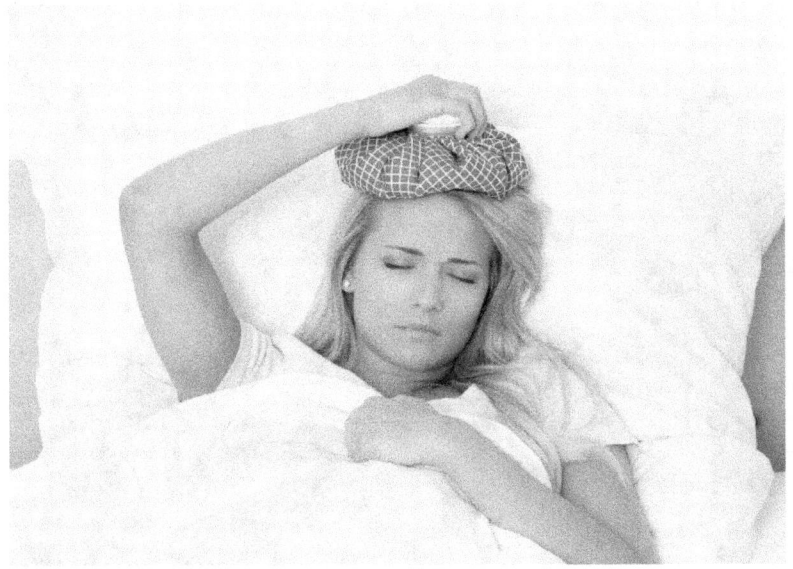

Ingredients:

- Very hot water, as needed
- 5 drops rosemary essential oil
- Clean cotton cloth

Instructions:

1. Fill a medium bowl with very hot water.
2. Add the rosemary essential oils and stir gently.
3. Dip a folded cotton cloth into the hot water and wring out the excess.
4. Place the compress over your eyes and forehead.
5. Let the compress set until it cools to body temperature.

6. Repeat the process three to five times or until your migraine subsides.

Antiseptic Surface Spray

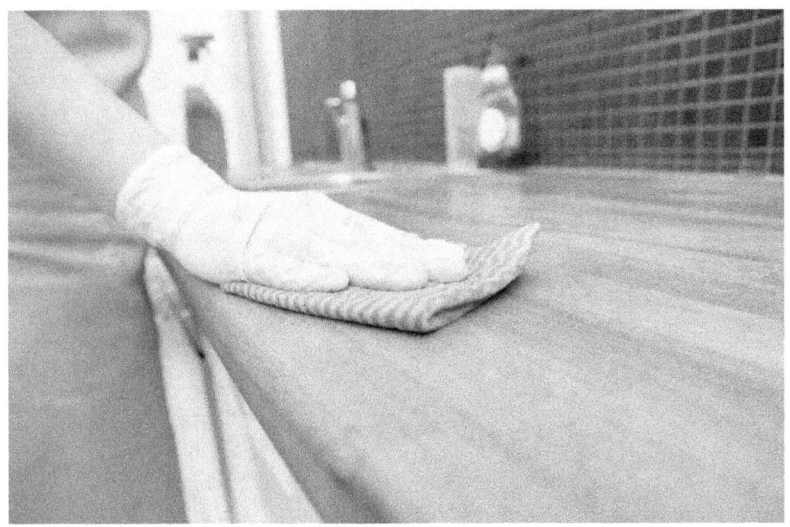

Ingredients:

- Empty 16-ounce plastic spray bottle
- 7 ounces distilled white vinegar
- 7 ounces filtered water
- 8 drops tea tree essential oil
- 6 drops lemon essential oil
- 6 drops bergamot essential oil

Instructions:

1. Add the essential oils to the empty plastic bottle.
2. Pour in the vinegar and water.
3. Shake the bottle gently to combine the ingredients.
4. Spray the liquid onto kitchen counters, cabinets, refrigerator shelves, and other surfaces.

5. Wipe the surface clean with a damp cloth or sponge.

All-Natural Lemon Furniture Polish

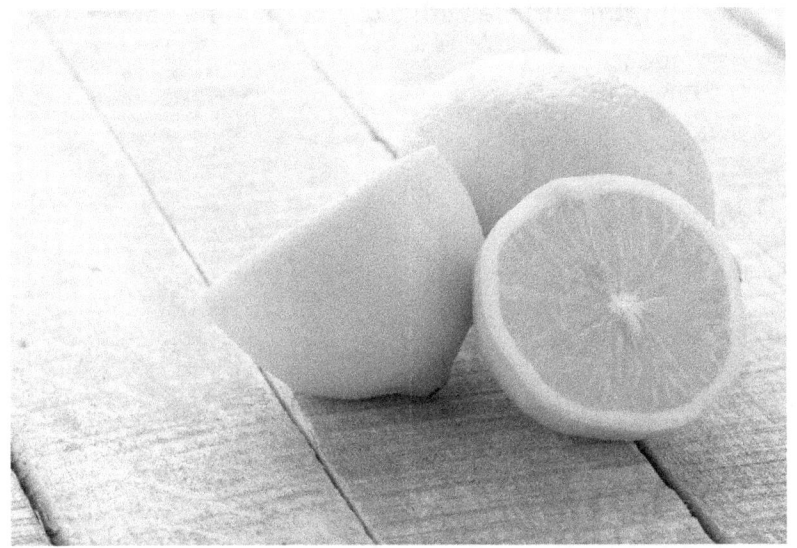

Ingredients:

- Empty 16-ounce plastic spray bottle
- 8 ounces extra-virgin olive oil
- 4 ounces distilled white vinegar
- 24 drops lemon essential oil
- Filtered water

Instructions:

1. Combine the olive oil, vinegar and lemon essential oil in the spray bottle.
2. Shake the bottle gently to combine the ingredients.
3. Fill the bottle the rest of the way with filtered water and shake again.

4. Spray the polish directly onto your furniture or a rag and rub it in.
5. Buff the surface with a dry cloth immediately after application.

Lavender Citrus Linen Spray

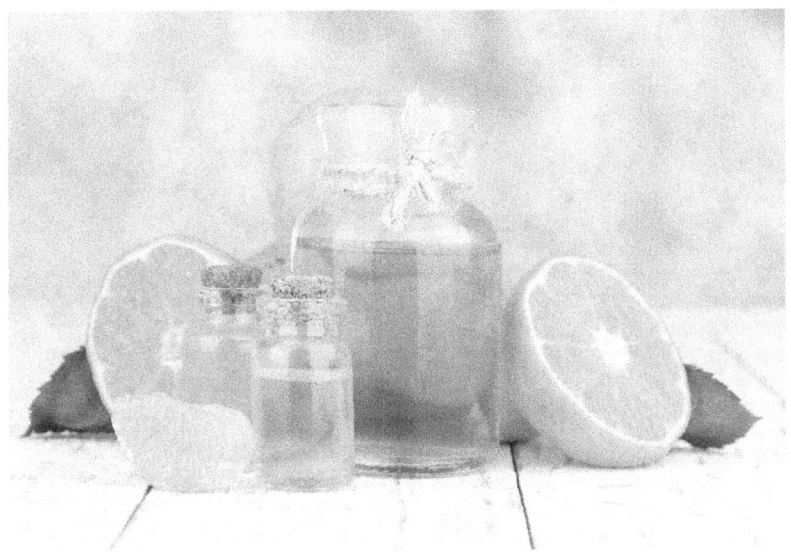

Ingredients:

- Empty 16-ounce plastic bottle
- ¾ cups organic hydrosol
- ¼ cup high-proof vodka
- 6 drops lavender essential oil
- 3 drops lemon essential oil
- 3 drops orange essential oil

Instructions:

1. Combine the hydrosol and vodka in the spray bottle.
2. Add the essential oil and shake the bottle gently to combine the ingredients.

3. Spritz the mixture onto pillows, mattresses, couches, and other fabric surfaces to freshen.

Citrus-Scented Carpet Deodorizer

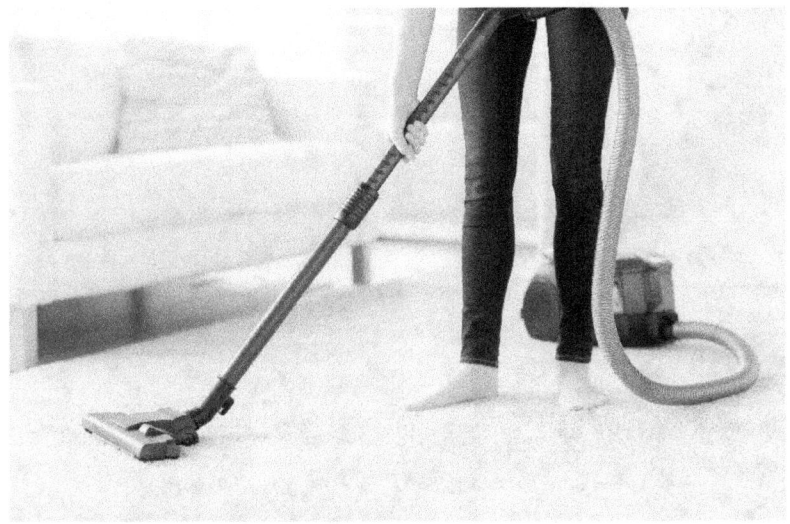

Ingredients:

- 1 cup baking soda
- 12 drops mandarin essential oil
- 10 drops lemongrass essential oil
- 6 drops ginger essential oil

Instructions:

1. Pour the baking soda into a medium-sized bowl.
2. Add the essential oils and stir well to combine.
3. Sprinkle the mixture over your carpet and let it sit for 30 minutes.
4. Vacuum your carpet as usual to remove odors.

Garbage Disposal Cleaning Cubes

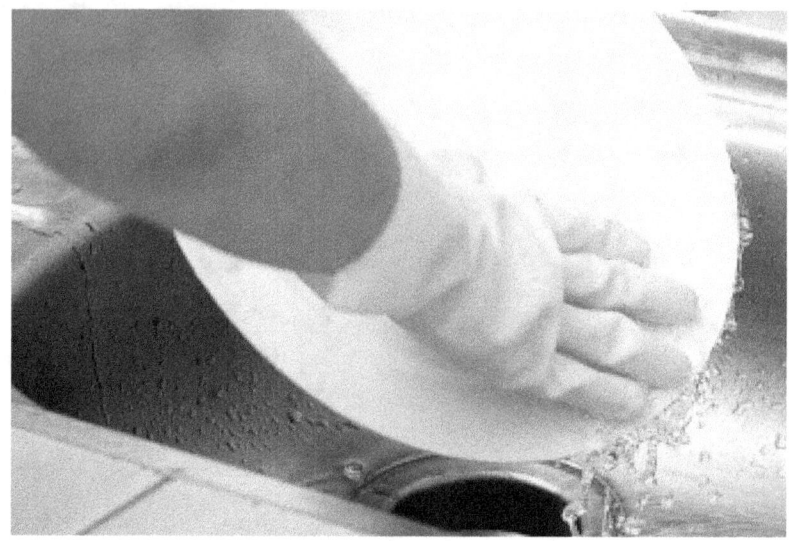

Ingredients:

- 1 ripe lemon, chopped
- 1 cup baking soda
- 1 cup coarse salt
- 1 tablespoon tea tree essential oil
- 1 tablespoon lemon essential oil

Instructions:

1. Place the lemons in a food processor and blend until pureed.
2. Add the baking soda and salt and pulse into a wet paste.
3. Blend in the essential oils until well combined.

4. Spoon the mixture into a flexible ice cube tray, filling the cubes evenly.
5. Set the ice cube tray out to dry for at least 24 hours.
6. Remove the cubes and store them in an airtight container.
7. To use the cubes, drop one cube into the garbage disposal while the water is running.

Lavender Tea Tree Laundry Soap

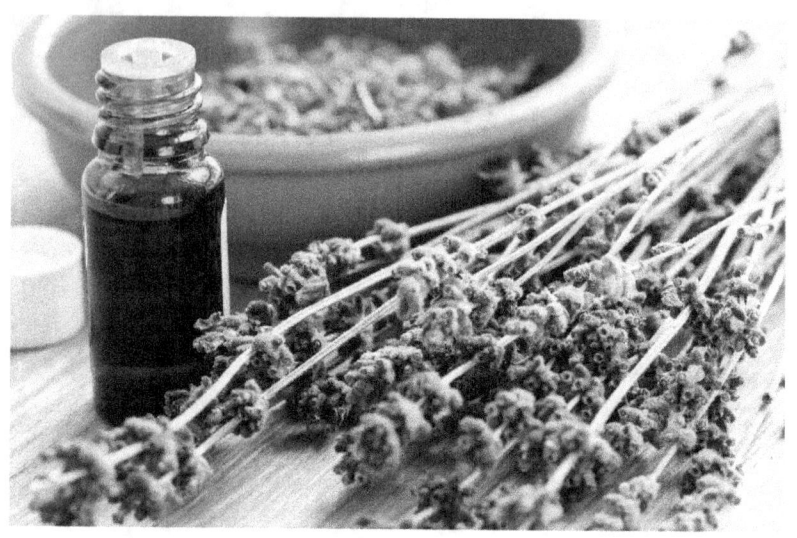

Ingredients:

- 1 bar of castile soap, unscented
- 2 cups borax
- 2 cups washing soda
- 2 teaspoons lavender essential oil
- 2 teaspoons tea tree essential oil
- 1 teaspoon lemon essential oil

Instructions:

1. Grate the bar of soap into a bowl.
2. Stir in the borax, washing soda, and essential oils until well combined.
3. Store the laundry soap in a glass jar or airtight container.

4. To use, add up to ¼ cup of laundry soap to a normal-sized load of laundry.

Antiseptic Floor Cleaner

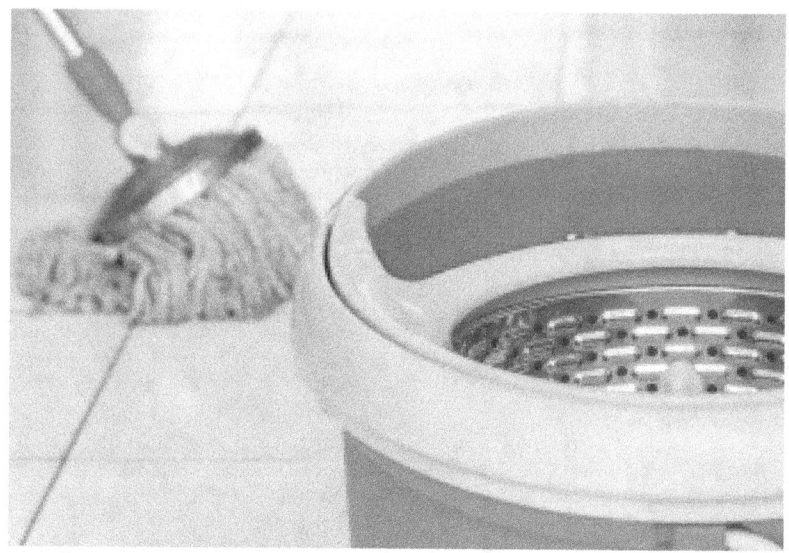

Ingredients:

- 2 tablespoons liquid castile soap, unscented
- 10 drops lemon essential oil
- 6 drops tea tree essential oil
- 4 drops bergamot essential oil
- 1 gallon warm water

Instructions:

1. Whisk together the soap and essential oils in a small bowl.
2. Fill a mop bucket with 1 gallon of warm water.
3. Add the soap mixture and stir until well combined.
4. Clean the floor with the warm water using a mop or sponge.

Conclusion

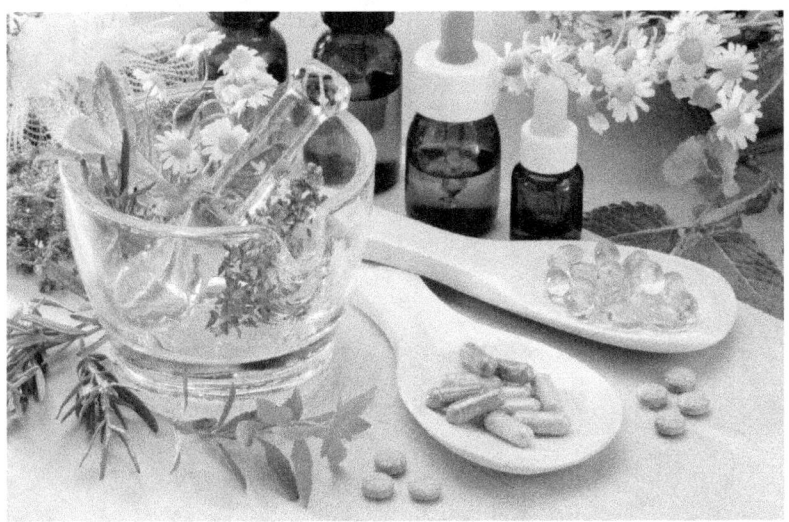

Essential oils are an important aspect of natural remedies and alternative medicine because they contain a wide variety of beneficial properties. Not only can essential oils provide health benefits for various diseases or conditions, but they can also be used in all-natural beauty products and cleaning supplies. By the time you finish this book you will have a firm understanding of how essential oils can be used for different purposes. If you are ready to experience the benefit of essential oils for yourself, pick a recipe and give it a try!